Methadone and Pregnancy

2nd Edition

By Travis Nevels

How Addiction Works

Opium is the liquid that comes from poppy seed pods, and has been cultivated by humans for around for 7000 thousand years. Modern day chemistry isolated the key ingredient in the poppy seed pod, and today we know it as morphine. Later morphine was manipulated to create codeine and heroin, and they are known as semi-synthetics. A purely synthetic opioid, which is not synthesized from opium or any other plant based material, is methadone. Methadone is a pure synthetic opioid.

The driving force behind heroin and opioid pain pills is the intensity of the "high" it creates. These addictive drugs force the brain to manufacture natural brain chemicals which are already made by the brain, and in fact are necessary for survival and normal mental functioning. The word endorphin is a short word for "endogenous morphine." Endogenous means inside or within the body. Morphine, as we know is chemical that has the potential for pain relief. When we receive a serious injury endorphins are released to block and diminish the feeling of pain. This also occurs when we take opioid based pain pills or heroin. These opioid substances are converted into morphine in the body, thus drenching our receptors with morphine. And, we like it, it feels good. Many of us are known to take opioids repeatedly and in large amounts; way beyond what a doctor would prescribe.

Another thing that happens however, is the brain senses an overload of endorphins, and to protect itself it stops producing endorphins on its own, or at least produces very little.

In addition, opioids stimulate the brain to manufacture naturally occurring neurotransmitters such as dopamine and serotonin.

Dopamine is a neurochemical that the brain makes on its own to make us feel good. When we eat something sweet, or watch a movie, fall in love, or have sex the brain rewards us with a small dose of dopamine. This is what we experience as pleasure.

The high that drug abusers experience comes from a large dose of morphine which attaches to a large number opiate receptors, also known as mu receptors. When endorphins (morphine) attaches to the mu receptors, they're hyper stimulated to produce Dopamine. Our brains produce Dopamine naturally, but not in the extreme high volumes that opioids force our brains to make.

Finally, there is another neurotransmitter called Serotonin, which is known as a mood elevator. When the brain produces Serotonin naturally, we feel better, and our mood improves. Things that stimulate Serotonin production includes exercise, eating food, having sex, walking in the sunshine, eating bananas, or listening to music. The activities that stimulate Serotonin are typically the same as those that stimulate Dopamine.

So with heavy opioid usage the brain is loaded up with endorphins, Dopamine, and Serotonin. It's no wonder we enjoy it so much. However, it's not natural. It's like putting jet engine on a child's bike. Just as the jet engine will over drive and wear out the bike; heavy opioid use wears out the mu receptors and other supporting structures in the brain. The brain can be said to burn out. And, as the brain attempts to protect itself, it shuts down many of the mu receptors. The brain can't shut all of them down because they're necessary for normal functioning. However, with an ever *decreasing* number of active mu receptors, the drug abuser has to take more and more of a drug to get the brain to process the heavy load of neurochemicals that the user needs to get high. The problem is that the high eventually becomes unachievable, and the user starts taking the drugs just to push back the feelings of withdrawal.

How Methadone Works

Heroin, morphine, and other opioids are fast acting drugs. When they lock into a mu receptor they deliver a powerful punch of chemical activity, and they're used up in a short period of time. Not only are these neurochemicals fast acting, they are also broken down and metabolized quickly by the liver. This is why the high is usually of such a short duration. This keeps an addict constantly on the move to re-up.

Methadone is a different kind of opioid in that it's slow acting. It moves onto the field of mu receptors slowly, and it takes a long time for methadone to be deactivated and metabolized by the liver. Methadone also delivers a trickle of stimulation to the mu receptors, but it's quite puny in comparison to heroin and morphine. It is unlikely that methadone give someone the sensation of being high since the activity is so slow and very weak in its delivery. For those who take too much methadone, the normal result is feeling drowsy or going to sleep. Most patients, who take too much methadone, voluntarily request a dose reduction.

Methadone has another excellent quality however. Methadone, once taken will lock in to the mu receptors, thus blocking any new opioids that might be taken later, as any new opioids won't be able to hook up. This is known as the blocking effect.

Opioid Addiction

Once a person reaches the point where they need the opioids just to function, and no longer get high from using, or just use to avoid the feelings of withdrawal, they've crossed the threshold into addiction.

The National Institute on Drug Abuse now defines addiction as "a chronic relapsing disease that is characterized by compulsive drug seeking and use, despite harmful consequences."

Let's analyze this definition. The National Institute on Drug Abuse defines addiction as a chronic (life-long) relapsing disease. If this definition is true, then addicts will relapse repeatedly throughout their lives. Have you relapsed before? How many times?

In my practice as a Counselor, I see that this definition is predominantly accurate. Almost all of my patients have relapsed several times, and that's why many choose to remain on methadone indefinitely. Many of them tell me, "I know methadone is safe, and it keeps me out of trouble and it allows me to keep money in my pocket, so I just want to stay on it."

In addition, the above definition defines addiction as a disease. Like anyone with a disease, they usually need to be treated by medical professionals. It's much like someone with diabetes who needs to monitor their blood sugar, so they can then take the correct amount of insulin in order to function normally. The same holds true for methadone patients, in that they need to monitor their withdrawal and craving symptoms resulting from opioid addiction, in order to take the correct amount of methadone, so they can function normally.

Ongoing methadone maintenance reduces the probability of relapsing and also allows patients to find and hold a job, stay out of jail, avoid disease, go to college, start businesses, and raise families. Methadone can do this because it eliminates cravings and also eliminates withdrawals.

A low to moderate dose of methadone can eliminate withdrawals; however it takes a larger dose to eliminate cravings. The "right" dose level is known as the therapeutic dose level or the stable dose level, and it's different for every patient.

The therapeutic dose level is determined by the patient. When a patient starts taking methadone they're started on a relatively low dose. This is because the prescribing doctor needs to be medically safe, and doesn't really know what opioids have been taken within the last few hours once a new patient comes into the clinic for the first time. Day by day however, as the patient comes to the clinic, they should be requesting dose increases until they find their own stable dose level.

Studies show that those who are addicted to opioids, and participate In methadone treatment are healthier, have reduced mortality, are more likely to be employed, and less likely to be incarcerated than those who do not.

Knowing this, wouldn't it make better sense for a pregnant patient to be in methadone treatment, rather than using street drugs?

Since methadone eliminates cravings and withdrawals (when taken at the therapeutic dose level), it also eliminates drug seeking behaviors. When a heavy drug abuser needs a "fix" they will often do illegal things to get the money they need, to buy the drugs they need. Many of these behaviors are unsafe, often invite violence, and increase the risk of incarceration. Do these behaviors sound healthy and safe for a mother to be, or an unborn child?

Other risky behaviors invite exposure to diseases and the spread of diseases like Hepatitis-B, Hepatitis-C, HIV, and STD's. Does the potential for exposure to these diseases sound like a healthy lifestyle for a mother to be, or an unborn baby?

Pregnant drug users also run the risk of contracting other well known street-drug associated diseases such as bacterial endocarditis, septicemia, tetanus, and cellulitis.

By eliminating withdrawals and cravings for opioids, methadone indirectly eliminates drug seeking behaviors which in turn will create a safer pregnancy, and the chances for a normal healthy delivery.

The short answer is yes, it's safe. Methadone treatment has been around since the1960's. Studies show that the longer someone stays in methadone treatment the better their outcome in terms of improved overall health, superior nutrition, avoidance of incarceration, and reduced exposure to diseases.

Researchers have found that those who participate in methadone treatment have no adverse effects on a person's ability to function normally.

Studies have shown that those who participate in methadone treatment are no different than the general population in their ability to learn and focus.

Methadone patient's also display normal motor skills and reaction times when compared to the general population.

Its common knowledge that illicit drug use leads to poor nutrition, since any money acquired is spent on drugs first. Meals are often skipped as the drug user continues to seek money for drugs. When a drug abuser finally does eat, they usually have very little money left over, and settle for a cup of coffee and a bag of chips. Does this sound like a healthy nutritious diet for a growing fetus? Where are the vitamins and minerals necessary for a healthy fetus with such a diet?

A stable dose of methadone contributes to a stable lifestyle. Once a patient become stable they can focus their energy on visiting local food pantries, acquiring food stamps, and seeking other assistance. Or, they can find employment.

A person cannot detox themselves off of illicit drugs by weaning themselves down. A heroin user who uses a gram a day, cannot follow a plan of using a gram a day for a week, and then three quarters of a gram a day for the next week, and the one half a gram a day for another week, and so forth. Why? Street drugs are impure and unregulated by the FDA (Food and Drug Administration). Street drugs are manufactured in dirty factories and the product can be cut with things like bleach, fertilizer, and even rat poison; anything to stretch the profits. It's no wonder drug users have so many skin infections at the injection site, endocarditis, collapsed veins, unspecified infections, and other medical challenges faced by exposure to unknown toxins. In the street, a gram bag of heroin one day does not equal a gram bag the next day, even though they may weigh the same. The purity is different from batch to batch and from supplier to supplier.

The same is true of pain pills. One day a drug dealer may have 10 mg Oxy's, and the next day he has 15 mg Percocet's. How does someone taper their dose down, in a controlled fashion, with such a mixed bag of pills?

I was told by one of my clients that a handful of pills might last a day, but a handful of heroin would last 30 minutes. And, this goes back to the definition of addiction, which states an addict has "uncontrolled usage." This means all drugs acquired will be consumed. Once the drugs are in hand, there is no plan, other than the immediate consumption of the entire quantity. There is no plan of using a little today, and putting some of it up in a vault for safe keeping, only to use a little tomorrow, and then a little the next day.

Methadone on the other hand, is kept in a vault, and is managed by medical professionals. The manufacture of methadone is regulated by the FDA and also monitored by the DEA (Drug Enforcement Agency) and several other national and state agencies.

Methadone is manufactured to be safe, and has been manufactured since 1939.

For that matter, pain pills are also manufactured to be safe, and are also subject to governmental oversight and regulation. However, opioid based pain pills are intended to be taken according to a doctor's prescription, just like methadone. However, as we know, drug abusers take pain pills according to their own wishes and desires. Many people take pain pills in very large quantities and they often use a grab bag of different pill types.

Methadone is different in that it's precisely dispensed. Methadone can be delivered according to very specific dose requirements. In this way a patient's dose level can be gradually increased in a controlled manner, and the doses can also be gradually decreased in controlled manner.

Based on studies in the 1960's and 1970's methadone treatment was recommended for pregnant opioid for patients. In 1997 the National Institute of Health Consensus Panel recommended methadone treatment as the standard of care for opioid addicted pregnant patients.

In 1973 the Food and Drug Administration recommended that all opioid addicted pregnant women go through a 21 day detox in order to be accepted into a federally licensed methadone treatment program. After further study however the FDA reversed their decision, sighting diminished fetal outcomes related to opioid withdrawal.

This book contains health care information, not medical advice.

Methadone and Body Weight and Metabolism

Heroin is a fast acting opioid in the body and it's also metabolized very quickly. That's why the high associated with heroin starts quickly and ends soon after. Methadone however moves onto the field of receptors more slowly, and peaks after about 3 hours of ingestion. It then lingers and is fully metabolized approximately 26 hours after ingestion. Because methadone remains "in play" for so long it's a good drug choice to block the effects of heroin and other illicit opiods for an extended period of time.

The therapeutic dose level for methadone tends to be related to a person's body and weight and tolerance for opiods. Body weight is somewhat of a judge of person overall blood volume. Bigger people have more blood than smaller people, and tend to need more methadone.

As the growing fetus adds more overall weight to the mother, she often needs to increase her therapeutic dose level.

There are those who are known to be fast metabolizers of methadone. The primary enzymes for breaking down methadone are known as the P540 enzyme system, and some people have more of it than others. For those with more P540 enzymes the quicker they metabolize methadone. Fast metabolizers have no relationship to body weight. Fast metabolizers can often benefit from a "spit-dose" of methadone whereby they take a dose in the morning and then take home another dose for later in the day.

Some studies have shown that a larger single daily dose of methadone affects the behavior of the fetus to a noticeable degree; whereas two smaller split doses, taken several hours apart on a given day, presents a more stable pattern of fetal behavior.

Overdose Potential and Other Concerns

If a person has been on heroin, pain pills, or street drugs for a long time, their drug tolerance is very high, and that's why they need to take a large amount of drugs to get high or get the relief they're looking for. When a person completely detoxes off of drugs, and lives an abstinence based lifestyle, their drug tolerance becomes very low. With a low drug tolerance, should a former addict relapse and take even a small amount of drugs, it can be deadly, and it can also cause a spontaneous abortion.

Can a person overdose on methadone? Yes, if you take enough of any drug you can overdose. The chances are not likely however with methadone, as your dose is regulated by the medical staff at your clinic. However, if you take home doses, and use benzo's, and/or alcohol, your chances of overdosing go way up, along with the chances of a spontaneous abortion. If you stop taking methadone for a time, then your tolerance for it will be decreased. To begin taking methadone again, and to be safe, you will need to start off with a low dose and work your way back up to a therapeutic level.

Methadone is not harmful to a person's immune system. Several studies show that opioid addicted women with serious diseases like HIV, Hepatitis-B, and Hepatitis-C live longer and are healthier, than those who rely on street drugs.

You may be surprised to learn that methadone and heroin are non-toxic. Both can be dangerous however when taken in excess because they could cause an overdose. Methadone however is safer than heroin, because it's regulated, manufactured according to strict standards, and dispensed by medical personnel in controlled units. Heroin on the hand is often cut with harmful substances which can present long term health problems for both the mother and her unborn baby.

Heroin is often injected which presents additional medical risks for the mother and her unborn baby.

Methadone is such a slow acting opioid that injecting it doesn't give the user the high they're looking for. Most people who have injected methadone have reported feeling nothing, while others have reported a mild 10 second high that wasn't very good. Injecting methadone can also be medically risky.

Many do report a decreased interest in sex while on methadone.

Methadone is a pure drug, not like heroin which is known to have elusive "cuts."

In Case Of an Overdose

If you believe someone has overdosed on methadone or heroin, roll the person over to one side, so if they were to vomit it will drain out of the mouth. If they're on their back any vomitus could be choking hazard. Call 911 immediately and remain with the person.

If the paramedics arrive in time they can inject an antagonist, such as Naloxone which will counter the effects of the opioid.

Signs of an Overdose

*Drowsiness

* Cold, clammy, bluish skin, or bluish lips

* Reduced body temperature

* Slow breathing or no breathing

* Nausea and vomiting

* Small pin-point pupils (constricted pupils)

* Unconscious

Methadone Interactions with Other Drugs

There are medicines that interact with methadone. The following list of drugs is known to cause the liver to metabolize methadone more quickly. When this drug interaction occurs it's not uncommon for a patient to request a dose increase:

1) Phenytoin (Dilantin)

2) Rifampin

3) Ritonavir (Norwir)

4) Carbamazepin (Tegretol)

5) Neverpine (Virammune)

There are other drugs that slow down the metabolism of methadone. When such drugs are taken along with methadone the normal effects of methadone are increased somewhat. This is due to methadone being broken down and removed more slowly, as a result, the methadone effects linger a little longer.

Once a person becomes accustomed to the lingering effects, should the interacting drug be removed, it's possible that a person could experience withdrawals. These drugs include:

1) Fluvoxamine (Luvox)

2) Ketoconazole (Nizoral)

3) Cimetidine (Tagamet)

4) Amitriptyline (Elavil)

Other drug types act as opioid blockers, and block all opioid type drugs including methadone. If you're taking any of the following drugs, you SHOULD NOT TAKE METHADONE.

1) Naltrexone (Revia)

2) Tramadol (Ultram)

3) Pentazocine (Talwin)

The Triangle of Danger

Below is what I call the "Triangle of Danger." It's well documented that people die from the interaction of any two of the following drugs:

<u>Methadone and/or other Opioids</u> have sedative properties, in that they slow down or depress the central nervous system (CNS), which controls breathing, heart rate, and other bodily functions. Combining methadone or other opioids with other drug types that also depress the CNS, dramatically increases the sedating effect and the danger of an overdose.

Benzodiazepines' (Benzo's) are a class of anti anxiety drugs which also depress the central nervous system. (Examples: Ativan, Xanax, Klonopin, Valium, and others) Combining methadone or other opioids with benzo's is a recipe for death, overdose, and possibly a spontaneous abortion.

Alcohol is probably the most common sedative known to man. Alcohol also depresses the central nervous system. Combining alcohol with methadone or benzo's is another high risk scenario for death, overdose, or a spontaneous abortion.

Mixing these drugs is known to be dangerous and is a leading cause of death in the United States.

Mixing any two of the three above drug choices is hazardous. Combining three of the above drug choices is insane.

The results of mixing these drugs in various combinations and strengths can lead to a person's CNS being so depressed that they get sleepy and lay down. They fall asleep and their breathing rate slows down. The reticular formation located in the brainstem regulates the reparatory drive, and when it becomes sedated or depressed as a result of drug use, it no longer functions to keep us breathing properly. The result is that an overdosed victim eventually stops breathing, becomes unconscious, slips into a coma, and eventually dies due to the lack of oxygen.

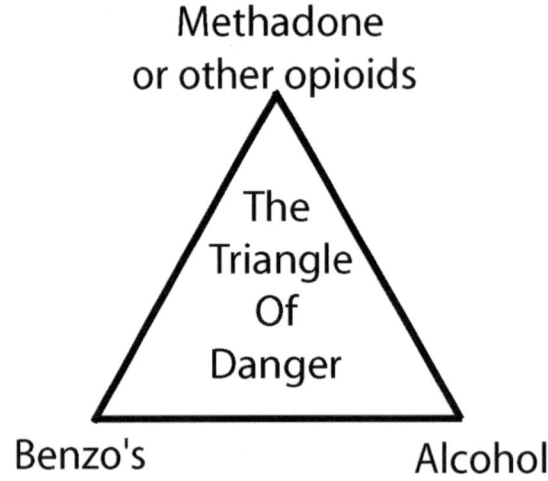

Women and Methadone

While taking methadone a woman can conceive, have a normal pregnancy, and also have a normal delivery.

Some women report having skipped periods or stop having periods while on methadone; however there are many other reasons that could cause this. For example, a woman could stop having her periods because:

- She is pregnant
- She is malnourished
- She has started menopause
- She is under stress
- She is on other medications
- She has other medical conditions

However, a woman can still get pregnant even without the presentation of a normal period.

It is a myth that methadone will not allow a woman to conceive. This is simply not true. I have seen several pregnancies in my clinic from women who have been on methadone for years.

Methadone treatment is the treatment of choice for opioid dependent patients who are pregnant.

Methadone and pregnancy has been extensively studied.

Pregnant patients who dose at their therapeutic dose level provide a comfortable and stress reduced environment for the developing baby.

Methadone treatment can avert premature labor, fetal distress, and diminish the likelihood of a miscarriage.

Decreasing your methadone dose during your first trimester can increase the chances of a miscarriage. It is strongly advised that you remain at your therapeutic dose level throughout your pregnancy.

A significant dose reduction could bring on withdrawal symptoms for you and your developing baby.

Consult with the medical staff at your clinic should you feel the need to increase your dose, which is normal during pregnancy.

Methadone has *not* been shown to cause fetal abnormalities.

Premature deliveries have been linked to cigarette smoking and poor nutrition, but not to methadone.

Low birth weight deliveries have been linked to cigarette smoking and poor nutrition, but not methadone.

Methadone dependent mothers will likely give birth to methadone dependent babies; however these babies can be safely weaned off methadone without harmful consequences.

At the time of this writing, the United States prison system does not widely administer methadone treatment to the incarcerated population, however some do. Of those that do, many "only" administer methadone to pregnant opioid dependent prisoners. This must be an indication that some prison systems recognize the benefits of methadone treatment for their pregnant opioid dependent inmates and their developing babies.

It is recommended that a pregnant woman terminate cigarette smoking, as cigarettes have been shown to cause medical challenges for the fetus, the delivery, and the health of the newborn.

Note that early signs of pregnancy, such as nausea and fatigue are often mistakenly thought to be withdrawal symptoms.

Find a Primary Care Doctor

It is important to a mother's general health, and the health of her developing baby to have prenatal and postnatal care. It is often true that methadone patients are reluctant to tell their primary care doctor that they're taking methadone, however it critically important with a pregnancy that you do so. You must *not* have your primary care doctor conducting medicine in the dark. Your doctor must be fully informed. This is vitally important for the mother's health and the health of the baby. Can you imagine a doctor prescribing medicine that has negative interaction with methadone? What kind of damage could that cause for the mother or the baby?

Imagine a mother choosing *not* to inform her doctor that she is taking methadone, and then there is a complication with the pregnancy. The mother might be charged with child abuse since she willfully withheld the truth of her methadone usage. This could result in legal problems and also the involvement of DSS (Department Of Social Services).

Imagine during delivery, a doctor prescribing an anti-anxiety pill to help relax a pregnant patient, only to learn afterwards she's on methadone. As we already discussed, methadone is known to negatively interact with benzodiazepines. Remember the "Triangle of Danger?"Methadone, when combined with benzo's can prove harmful to the mother and the baby.

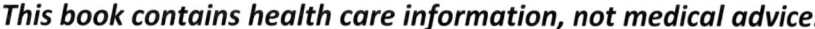

Imagine a doctor prescribing an opioid based pain pill, and doing so completely unaware of a pregnant patient's methadone usage.

Can you imagine a pregnant patient currently participating in methadone treatment, and going to the hospital to deliver her baby and *not* informing the medical staff that she is on methadone? This would certainly be medically unsafe, but could also result in criminal charges for the mother.

Know that it is illegal for your methadone clinic to communicate with your primary care doctor, without your written consent to do so. It is advised that you provide the written consent, so your primary care doctor and your methadone clinic can freely communicate and coordinate your medical care. Your clinic will provide the necessary consent forms.

This book contains health care information, not medical advice.

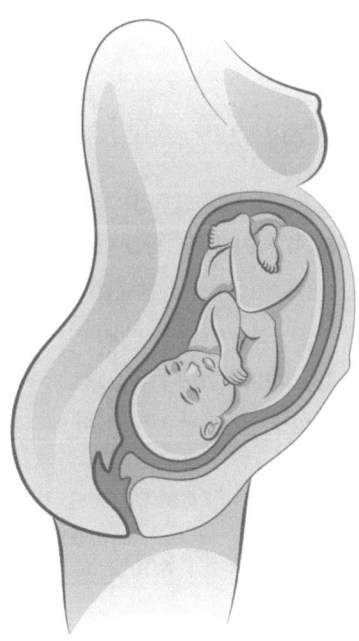

Goals During Pregnancy

- Involvement in prenatal care and postnatal care
- Good nutritional support
- Minimize fetal exposure to dangerous drugs
- Remain on a therapeutic dose level of methadone
- Locate a stable and safe living environment
- Avoid risky behaviors
- Participation in a drug recovery program
- Regular visits with your primary doctor
- HIV and Hepatitis testing
- Counseling regarding post-partum depression
- Getting adequate sleep
- Drinking plenty of water
- Aerobic exercise and stretching exercises
- Stop smoking
- No alcohol
- No illicit drug use
-

Methadone Treatment as Related to Pregnancy

It is well documented that opioid use puts a pregnancy at risk. Heroin and methadone mothers deliver higher rates of fetal still births, as well as baby's with low birth weight, small head circumference, growth retardation, and neonatal death as compared to non-opioid using mothers. However, methadone babies report higher birth weights and larger head circumference than heroin exposed babies. Even though methadone exposed babies tend to have lower birth weights, they are usually within normal ranges.

Babies exposed to methadone in utero usually have normal mental and physical development.

Intravenous heroin users place a baby at risk for bacterial infections from needle contamination.

Shared needles may be cleaned with bleach which can reduce the transmission of HIV, however bleach is not as effective against the Hepatitis-B nor the Hepatitis-C viruses.

A rapid detox or a cold turkey detox from heroin or methadone will put heavy stress on the mother and the fetus and could cause a spontaneous abortion.

Rather than detox, it would be best for a pregnant heroin user to begin treatment at a methadone clinic as soon as possible.

A pregnant methadone patient should *not* detox or wean herself off of methadone, but rather plan on remaining in treatment for the remainder of her pregnancy. Once the baby is delivered she can consider detoxing if she chooses.

Babies born to opioid addicted mothers are more likely to be premature and/or small at birth, as compared to babies born to non-opioid addicted mothers. Such neonates often have problems related to breathing, eating, infection, and may be prone to SIDS (Sudden Infant Death Syndrome).

Babies exposed to opioids including methadone may experience withdrawal symptoms after birth. Such symptoms can include: poor feeding patterns, vomiting, diarrhea, tremors, sneezing, sweating, high pitched crying, and restlessness. This grouping of symptoms is known as Neonatal Abstinence Syndrome (NAS).

Not every opioid exposed baby will experience NAS, however the rate of NAS according to some studies is around 50%, while other studies indicate higher rates of occurrence.

NAS usually begins soon after birth, and some present the most severe withdrawal symptoms 72 hours after birth. In some cases these symptoms can be addressed with a methadone solution by mouth or feeding tube.

Untreated NAS can lead to neonatal seizures and in extreme cases death.

Babies who experience NAS do not generally report any deficits in intelligent testing later in life.

A mother's increase in methadone usage during pregnancy does *not* statistically correlate to an increase in a newborn's severity of NAS.

Pregnant women, who are addicted to opioids, and make the commitment to abandon the lifestyle of chasing street drugs, and choose instead to enter methadone treatment, tend to become more stable. Once they're stable on methadone, they have the chance to get their life back on track. Many are able to find the time to go to their doctor for prenatal care, which increases the health of the mother and the baby. Prenatal care also increases the chances of a successful delivery and an overall healthier baby.

With stability, a pregnant patient can improve her diet which will add weight to the baby.

Once a pregnant woman gives up street drugs, and begins methadone treatment, she has the opportunity to gain some steadiness in her life. She has the chance to eliminate drug seeking behaviors, and as a result of her new lifestyle, she can find more time for sleep. Quality sleep for 7- 8 hours per night is critical for the health of the mother and her unborn baby.

Alcohol and Pregnancy

According the The Department of Health, if you're pregnant you should avoid alcohol altogether. If however you do drink, they recommend that a pregnant woman limit her intake of alcohol to one or two small glasses of wine once or twice a week only.

When a pregnant woman drinks, the alcohol travels to the fetus by way of the mother's blood, through the placenta to the baby. A baby's liver is known to be one of the last organs to mature. If a younger fetus were to be exposed to alcohol, there could be serious developmental problems.

Any alcohol exposure for the developing baby can affect the outcome.

It is during the first 3 months of development that a baby is at the greatest risk for developing problems resulting from alcohol exposure. During this time frame alcohol has been linked to miscarriage, birth abnormalities, premature birth, and low birth weight.

Babies exposed to alcohol during the second half of pregnancy have been shown to have an increased risk for learning difficulties and behavioral problems.

Heavy drinking throughout pregnancy can cause the baby to have Fetal Alcohol Syndrome (FAS). Babies with FAS are characterized as having restricted growth, facial abnormalities, along with behavioral and learning disabilities.

> Binge drinking, which can loosely be defined as heavy drinking on occasional bases, has been shown to affect newborns. Binge drinking has been linked to milder forms of FAS.

Cigarette Smoking and Pregnancy

Cigarette smoking during pregnancy presents its own set of risks. Nicotine and other harmful chemicals such as lead, carbon monoxide, ammonia, and tar, are known to constrict blood vessels. These substances are known as "vasoconstrictors". As cigarette chemicals attach themselves to the lining of the blood vessels, the blood vessels react to these irritants by constricting, and thus reducing blood flow. The heart reacts by increasing pumping pressure, because it takes more effort to pump blood though smaller "pipes." Hypertension (high blood pressure) is a problem for the mother and the developing baby.

Consider the blood supply being delivered to the developing baby by way of the umbilical cord, which contains two umbilical arteries. Now imagine the umbilical arteries being lined with irritating toxins. As those umbilical arteries constrict, less oxygen rich blood is delivered to the fetus.

Cigarette smoking during pregnancy is associated with premature delivery, low birth weight, and still births.

Exposure to cigarettes while in utero and after birth has been shown to present an increased risk for SIDS (Sudden Infant Death Syndrome) as well as ADHD.

Detoxing Off Methadone While Pregnant

In the vast majority of cases it is *not* a good idea to detox off of methadone during a pregnancy. The detox experience is unhealthy for the mother and the developing fetus.

According to the majority of studies, there is no relationship between the mother's methadone dose level during pregnancy, and the severity of the newborns withdrawal symptoms.

Should a pregnant patient demand a detox, it should be coordinated with an obstetrician or medical doctor who can monitor the mother and fetus during the detox time frame.

Detoxing off methadone has been shown to increase fetal distress.

Detoxification early in a pregnancy carries the potential of a spontaneous abortion.

Detoxification later in a pregnancy can be severe enough to induce a premature delivery.

A pregnant patient might choose to detox because she's moving to an area that does not have a methadone clinic. A pregnant patient in this situation should make every effort to remain on her stable dose level, and with her home clinic until the baby is delivered; then detox.

A pregnant patient might need to be removed from a clinic because of her disruptive and incompliant behaviors. In such a case, she should be transferred to another clinic if possible.

If you should find yourself pregnant, and being removed from your clinic against your will, you should try to control your behaviors, and attempt to negotiate a way to remain in treatment, or seek out another methadone clinic.

This book contains health care information, not medical advice.

Breast Feeding

A pregnant patient should work to remain stable on methadone, so she can remain healthy in regards to nutrition, psychological strength, adequate sleep, and the avoidance of risky behaviors. The result of a healthy lifestyle during pregnancy is a healthy delivery, of a healthy baby, by a healthy mother. A healthy mother is then able to breastfeed her newborn because she has the energy and nutritional support to do so.

Breastfeeding is always encouraged if possible as it increases the mother-baby psychological bond. Previous or ongoing methadone use by the mother does *not* change this.

Small amounts of methadone will likely pass from mother to baby, however methadone levels in breast milk is very low, and some studies claim it's so low that it does not affect or harm the baby.

Breastfeeding does not eliminate NAS, but some reports claim that it does lessen withdrawal symptoms.

To breastfeed, a mother needs to be stable in her recovery. A mother who is taking illicit drugs should *not* breastfeed due to the potential of exposing the neonate to various toxins and powerful drugs.

Mothers who abuse alcohol should *not* breastfeed.

Mothers with HIV should *not* breastfeed.

Methadone mothers are encouraged to breast feed, as this practice is best for the baby from a nutritional standpoint as well as for mother-baby bonding.

Breast feeding is deemed safe by the medical establishment for mothers who are participating in methadone treatment.

Babies born to methadone treated mothers may have withdrawal symptoms; however they can be weaned off methadone with no lasting effects.

Breast feeding is not safe for women who are HIV+, as the virus can pass from the mother to the child by way of breast milk.

Mothers with Hepatitis-B are *not* recommended to breastfeed, as the virus is present in breast milk, and can be passed along to the baby. The greatest risk for a newborn being exposed to Hepatitis-B is during the delivery process, which can bring the newborn into contact with infected blood.

A baby born to a Hepatitis-B positive mother will be treated with a vaccine. The Hepatitis-B vaccine is given soon after birth, and then there are two additional vaccinations given later. The Hepatitis-B vaccination stimulates the newborn to mount an immune response, by manufacturing antibodies that will be prepared to fight off an actual Hepatitis-B virus.

The Hepatitis-C virus is *not* found in breast milk, but it is present in blood. So, like the previous discussion of Hepatitis-B, the baby could be exposed to infected blood during the delivery process. Mothers with Hepatitis-C however can breastfeed. Note that if a mother's nipple was to be injured (possibly during breastfeeding), then the newborn should discontinue breast feeding since the infant could ingest the virus by taking in the mother's blood at the injured nipple site.

Also, if the mother were to supply milk by way of a breast pump, and have nipple trauma, then the presence of blood could be in the pumped milk. Therefore any milk in the pump must be discarded. Further, the pump itself must be destroyed or discarded. Once the nipple has fully healed, breastfeeding can resume.

Post-Partum Depression (PPD)

Post Partum Depression (PPD) is a common occurrence with many pregnancies. It's not well understood, however some have suggested it may be related to hormonal changes as a woman's body returns to its non-pregnant state. Common complaints for PPD include fatigue, anxiety, irritability, sadness, a reduced interest in sex, unexplained crying episodes, disruptive sleeping patterns, and a decline in self care.

Once the baby is born, the woman is often left alone with the difficult task of caring for the baby, while she herself is recovering from the delivery.

Women who have a history of depression appear to be more susceptible to PPD.

Women who have substance abuse issues are also more susceptible to PPD.

For women with substance abuse problems, the risk of relapsing during a PPD episode increases dramatically. This is a situation that any drug abuser and their family should be made aware of and be sensitive to.

Many women who experience PPD do not recognize it as PPD, and may lash out at family members or blame negative life events as a reason to be upset, and possibly a reason to relapse.

Some women with PPD symptoms can struggle with mother-baby bonding.

If a woman develops PPD, she may blame it on methadone and determine she should detox immediately. This is *not* a good idea, because the likelihood of a relapse following the birth of her baby is extremely high. The mother-baby bond is important for long term physical and psychological development of the baby. Should the mother chose to detox, she will have to deal with withdrawal symptoms including, irritability, anxiety, headaches, insomnia, cravings, and a low threshold for stress. These symptoms do not contribute to mother-baby bonding, nor does it help a new mother give baths, change diapers, rock the baby, and care for herself. Raising and nurturing a newborn is a strain in itself without adding withdrawal symptoms into the mix.

During any detox, the withdrawal symptoms and the cravings can become difficult. Some new mothers who choose to detox may soon return to methadone treatment, which would be the preferred path. However, some may return to illicit drug use, and relapse. Such a situation would be a disaster for a newborn and the family. I have heard of mother's taking their newborn baby with them to make drug deals.

A relapse not only involves a return to illegal drug use, but also a return to drug seeking behaviors. Mothers who remain in methadone treatment however, are less likely to be incarcerated, are healthier, less stressed, get better sleep, and are better able to care for their newborn.

As with any type of depressive episode, many can benefit by getting more exercise, walking or stretching, getting more sunlight, eating better (bananas stimulate Serotonin production which is known to improve mood), meditating or praying, reading, going to church, getting more sleep, and socializing.

If PPD symptoms persist or become severe, see a doctor.

Storing Methadone

Always keep track of the number of methadone bottles you have and always keep them locked way in a lock box and out of the reach of young children. Remember, methadone is a powerful drug and could kill a child. NEVER give a child methadone.

Buprenorphine and Pregnancy

Methadone, heroin, and morphine are full agonist. An agonist turns on mu receptors (opiate receptors) in the brain. In fact these substances fire up the mu receptors so well that people get addicted to them.

Methadone is a weak agonist compared to heroin, morphine, and opium which are strong agonists. Think about it as a dimmer switch that regulates the light intensity of an overhead light. You can dial up the bulbs brightness or you can dial it down. If full-on brightness is like heroin then low intensity brightness would be more like methadone.

Buprenorphine is partial agonist which means they turn on mu receptors' but not as much full agonists.

Buprenorphine however has another quality. Buprenorphine is known to have a greater *affinity* for mu receptors than heroin, methadone, and morphine. This means its better able to seek out mu receptors and connect with them compared to drugs with a lower affinity. Buprenorphine has such a strong affinity for mu receptors they will kick out any opioid that may already be locked in. In other words, Buprenorphine cannot easily be blocked out. Heroin and methadone have less of an affinity for mu receptors compared to Buprenorphine. Therefore, Buprenorphine win out over most other drugs that compete for mu receptors. And, once Buprenorphine is coupled with a mu receptor, it cannot easily be dislodged. Buprenorphine is the big boy on the block.

Once Buprenorphine locks into a receptor, it will block out all comers. This is why Buprenorphine patients who inject heroin *don't* get high. When the heroin is introduced, there are little or no available receptors to bind to. Heroin likes to float in and find easy targets (mu receptors) to lock in to, but with Buprenorphine in place there are no easy receptors available, and heroin doesn't have the affinity to knock out any of the Buprenorphine molecules.

Buprenorphine is an excellent drug; however it is not generally recommended that a person switch off of methadone and onto Buprenorphine. In fact it would be dangerous to do so, especially for a pregnant patient. There must be a compelling medical reason to switch from methadone to Buprenorphine. Consult with your doctor for advice as to whether or not you might be a good candidate.

For methadone patients who wish to switch over to Buprenorphine, they first need to detox themselves off of methadone. Once they get their daily methadone dose down to 30 mgs (your clinic may vary), then they might can switch over to Buprenorphine immediately, or they might be required to wait 24 hours before starting Buprenorphine. This means a person might have to go cold turkey off of methadone for a day before starting their first dose of Buprenorphine. This can be a difficult time for any patient and certainly not a good idea for a pregnant patient, as it will add distress to the mother and the baby.

Buprenorphine needs to be introduced to an empty field of mu receptors in order to start off correctly. If there are mu receptors with opioid molecules in them, the Buprenorphine will kick those opioids out, and take over. The result will be precipitous withdrawal. In this scenario, Buprenorphine is said to *precipitate* withdrawal. This is because the mu receptors are being energized by a full agonist like heroin or methadone, but when Buprenorphine kicks them out, the brain will endure a rapid reduction in agonist activity. Remember Buprenorphine is only a partial-agonist. The result is like a brain with all the lights being dimmed at the same time, and the result is instant withdrawal.

I've known a few heroin addicts who thought they'd like to try Buprenorphine, and quickly went in to precipitous withdrawal. Some have told me it was the worst experience they ever went through as an addict. Of course, these people didn't know they would lose their buzz so quickly, and fall instantly into severe dope sickness – yuk! This is why Buprenorphine needs to be introduced to an empty field of mu receptors, *so it can take over and provide relief to a person who's already in withdrawal.*

When people come in to the clinic for the first time, and tell us they haven't had anything in a day or two, they're likely good candidates for Buprenorphine. Others may say they took a couple of Oxy's a few hours ago, and in most cases like this we would ask them to sign up today, but come back tomorrow to get their first dose.

If your pregnant and currently using street drugs, you need to consider the above information regarding Buprenorphine treatment. You'll need to be in withdrawal when you start Buprenorphine. Methadone is more forgiving in this regard. But, as always, check with the doctor at your clinic.

If you're pregnant and wanting to switch from methadone treatment to Buprenorphine treatment, remember first that you need a compelling medical reason to do so. However, assuming for the moment you have a compelling medical reason, know that you will have to "safely" detox yourself down to 30 mgs of methadone (your clinic may vary), and then possibly go cold turkey for 24 before starting Buprenorphine treatment. Such withdrawals are not healthy for the mother or the baby.

Check with the doctor at your clinic before you decide switch from methadone to Buprenorphine or vice versa.

Summary

If you're thinking about getting pregnant, it's advised that you be stable before you try and get pregnant. Your options include being stable on methadone, buprenorphine, or being drug free and stable. The preference of course would be that you're stable in an abstinence based recovery program. In this way the developing baby is never exposed to any illegal or potentially harmful substances.

The next best option for someone choosing to get pregnant would be that you're participating in methadone or buprenorphine treatment, and you're stable.

If you choose to get pregnant while you're stable, and participating in methadone or buprenorphine treatment, or abstinence based program, it is advised that you continue with your treatment modality throughout your pregnancy and beyond.

It's like the old saying goes, "Leave with the one who brought you."

The only twist to the above statement, is that if you're stable on Suboxone (Buprenorphine and Naloxone), and realize you're pregnant, it's usually advised that you switch to Subutex (Buprenorphine only). It's thought that exposing the fetus to two drugs; Buprenorphine as well as Naloxone, is an unnecessary risk. Most agree that it's best to keep the mother and baby stable on Buprenorphine, but eliminate the Naloxone component if possible. *However, speak with the doctor at your clinic to be sure.*

Finally, on the chance that you're still involved with street drugs when you realize you're pregnant, it's strongly advised that you seek methadone or buprenorphine treatment so you can get stable as soon as possible.

FDA Pregnancy Categories

The FDA has established five categories to indicate the potential of a drug to cause birth defects if used during pregnancy. The categories are determined by the reliability of documentation and the risk to benefit ratio. They do not take into account any risks from pharmaceutical agents or their metabolites in breast milk.

Note that Methadone, Buprenorphine, and Naloxone are all Category C drugs.

Category A - Adequate and well-controlled studies have failed to demonstrate a risk to the fetus in the first trimester of pregnancy (and there is no evidence of risk in later trimesters).

Category B - Animal reproduction studies have failed to demonstrate a risk to the fetus and there are no adequate and well-controlled studies in pregnant women.

Category C - Animal reproduction studies have shown an adverse effect on the fetus and there are no adequate and well-controlled studies in humans, but potential benefits may warrant use of the drug in pregnant women despite potential risks.

Category D - There is positive evidence of human fetal risk based on adverse reaction data from investigational or marketing experience or studies in humans, but potential benefits may warrant use of the drug in pregnant women despite potential risks.

Category X - Studies in animals or humans have demonstrated fetal abnormalities and/or there is positive evidence of human fetal risk based on adverse reaction data from investigational or marketing experience, and the risks involved in use of the drug in pregnant women clearly outweigh potential benefits.

Category N - FDA has not classified the drug.

SUMMARY

As we wrap up this little exploration into the possible twists and turns of pregnancy, I hope you have learned something meaningful along the way. The overriding concern is that once you determine you're pregnant, you must think about the health of the baby first and foremost at all times. If you're addicted to heroin or illicit opioids then you need to seek help at a methadone clinic as soon as possible. Clinics these days usually offer both methadone and buprenorphine treatment options. In addition, you need to find a doctor as soon as possible, as statistics show that prenatal medical attention results in better postnatal outcomes.

The overriding message that the current research tells us, is that if you're involved in methadone treatment and pregnant, you need to stay on methadone throughout your pregnancy and beyond. You can detox later when your child is older.

Or, if you're involved in buprenorphine treatment and you're pregnant, you need to stay on buprenorphine throughout your pregnancy and beyond. Again, you can detox later when your child is older.

Inform the doctor at your clinic as soon as you realize you're pregnant.

Request a pregnancy test at your clinic if you suspect you might be pregnant.

If you're still involved with street drugs and the associated behaviors, seek a methadone clinic as soon as possible. Street drugs and risky behaviors do not contribute to a healthy pregnancy.

And finally, knowing that a relapse can be very harmful for you and your baby, you must work that much harder to ensure you don't relapse, as you have the health of your child in your hands.

Resources

Alcoholics Anonymous - (212) 870-3400 - www.aa.org

Narcotics Anonymous - www.na.org

Cocaine Anonymous - www.ca.org

T3Publications.com

Made in the USA
Columbia, SC
25 July 2025